Improving Life for Thyroid Patients

Famous People with Thyroid Problems

© 2008 By: James M. Lowrance

INTRODUCTION

How much does thyroid disease affect the quality of life of those who suffer them? Is this really an important or worthwhile aspect to consider and address? In my belief as a Thyroid Patient Advocate being treated for autoimmune hypothyroidism and having corresponded with 1,000s of other patients with both hypothyroid and hyperthyroid conditions since 2003, I absolutely believe this to be an important aspect.

More education has become available in regard to thyroid disease in general over the past two decades and the quality-of-life for treated thyroid patients, deserves as much attention in my opinion as do aspects of diagnosis and treatment. Much of the public lacks understanding in the fact that thyroid disease patients can be greatly affected by their disease with symptoms of thyroid hormone imbalance affecting every part of their bodies and emotions.

Some patients are seriously affected by the life changing effects of thyroid disease and find it difficult to cope with symptoms and their reduced ability to carry on the same level of activity as before their disease onset.

Improving Life for Thyroid Patients

The U.S. National Institutes of Health is conducting a clinical trial studying thyroid patients in regard to their quality of life following treatments they are given to correct their disorders. The study entitled "Health-Related Quality of Life for Thyroid Patients", once completed will be published for review by the public and by those in the medical field. It will be interesting to see what is revealed in this survey involving patient-respondents.

In this book, I will be looking at different aspects of the effects thyroid disease has on its patients and at the importance of better optimized treatment and coping-methods that can help patients regain a better quality-of-life.

TABLE OF CONTENTS:

CHAPTER ONE: Are Thyroid Patients Complainers?

CHAPTER TWO: Men Get Thyroid Disease Too!

CHAPTER THREE: Famous Thyroid Disease Sufferers are Increasing Public Awareness

CHAPTER FOUR: Oprah Winfrey's Diagnosis of Hypothyroidism

CHAPTER FIVE: Thyroid Research Every Doctor Should Know

CHAPTER SIX: Thyroid Hormone Replacement and Antidepressants

CHAPTER SEVEN: Stress Management for Thyroid Patients

CHAPTER EIGHT: Anxiety and Depression in Thyroid Disease

CHAPTER NINE: My Experience with Thyroid Related Anxiety and Panic

CHAPTER TEN: More of My Personal Thyroid Story

CHAPTER ELEVEN: Treated Hypothyroidism and Weight Gain

CHAPTER TWELVE: Book Review for "Hypothyroidism Type 2"

CHAPTER THIRTEEN: Embracing Your Thyroid Disease?

CHAPTER ONE

Are Thyroid Patients Complainers?

You may see the heading of this chapter and wonder what in the world could this one be about?! My intention in this article is to bring attention to the fact that thyroid disease symptoms can be very serious and no matter who they may affect, they can seriously alter a person's life and have a negative impact upon their emotions and quality of life. This includes even the strongest of people out there who may experience the onset of a thyroid disease.

Over the years I have corresponded with fellow thyroid disease patients on forums and by e-mail, plus a few I've been in phone contact with or who I know in-person, who report that, friends or loved ones believe they are being complainers. In some cases this was devastating to the person because on top of severe symptom struggles and feeling at times as if they are barely surviving their disease, they have someone make such an inconsiderate and non-compassionate remark toward them.

I have read the testimonies of patients whose marriages crumbled due to the frustration of a spouse who thought their husband or wife was over-reacting to the symptoms of their disease or who were simply playing on their sympathy and trying to get attention.

If these people with this view that thyroid patients are over-reacting to their symptoms, could step into that person's shoes for just one day, they would gain a completely different understanding. Using myself for an example, previous to thyroid disease, I was never one to give in when I was sick or allow symptoms to keep me from doing the things I enjoyed, including putting in a hard days' work. I remember times working when I had severe flu symptoms, bronchitis and other times when I worked even when I thought I was suffering pneumonia. I made doctor visits probably less than once every five years and had to be very sick to see one and it usually required that my wife prompted me before I would make a doctor office visit.

I'm a big guy at 6 foot, 235 lbs and I have always been strong and love outdoors sports but the onset of thyroid disease hit me very hard and I basically buckled under the symptoms of it for a time.

I remember after going through a very stressful period of time, falling into incredibly harsh symptoms that in my case cycled between hypothyroid and hyperthyroid symptoms at first. I would experience incredibly severe fatigue and exhaustion and would then phase into extreme panic attacks with profuse sweating and temporary rapid weight loss. I lost my ability to concentrate and completely lost my appetite for several weeks at a time.

Fear of the unknown of what was happening to me, sunk me into a severe state of anxiety and depression, at which time, I finally went to see a doctor. The doctor incorrectly diagnosed me with emotional problems only and I had to demand blood testing before the proper diagnosis was made. Even with my treatment having been optimized since, I can occasionally fall into mild to moderate spells of symptoms and infrequently I can experience severe symptoms.

In my case I have a supportive and compassionate family who, have been supporting me from the beginning of my health problems. I truly wish all thyroid patients had this same benefit but sadly, some do not.

I know other strong people who have been seriously affected by thyroid disease symptoms, including a man I am in occasional communication with by phone whom also has hypothyroidism caused by Hashimoto's thyroiditis, as I do. He was previously a race car driver and has told me often of the fact that he seldom experienced fear on the track or otherwise in his life. This changed when he experienced the onset of thyroid disease and he has at times gone through serious struggles with the symptoms it has caused him. Famous athletes have experienced thyroid disease and have gone through severe struggles as well, until they were properly diagnosed and treated. This includes names like Carl Lewis, 10-time Olympic gold winner in track and field and Gail Devers, an Olympic sprinter who also won a gold medal in her sport.

If you are the spouse, loved one or friend of a thyroid disease patient, I appeal to you, to exercise patience, understanding and compassion toward the thyroid patients in your life. This can be greatly instrumental in helping them to benefit more from treatment and in coping with the disease that has greatly affected their lives.

CHAPTER TWO

Men Get Thyroid Disease Too!

It is a fact that thyroid disease in-general affects at least five times as many woman as men. Despite this fact, men from all walks of life, including professional athletes experience thyroid problems. Following below, is information I shared with a man who described to me symptoms he was experiencing from hypothyroidism. He was experiencing the typical under-active thyroid gland symptoms but the two of most concern to him were his emotional ones and his diminished libido (sex drive). Following below are some of the things I shared in response to him.

Quote: "The titration (dose adjustments) of your thyroid medication can take several changes over several months, before they get you to a good euthyroid (normal hormone level) state. It's hard to be "patient" with the process but we have no choice. Also, while you might be a patient that sees very good resolution of symptoms with thyroid hormone therapy, many of us have somewhat satisfactory relief but never reach 100% of what we were before experiencing the disease.

Improving Life for Thyroid Patients

I've had many improvements but still experience occasional fatigue, brain fog etc... These are much improved in many ways and less frequent, since being treated but have never been completely gone.

The libido problem should also improve for you over time. I almost completely lost interest in intimacy as well for a while when my symptoms were at their worst and before treatment. This is an embarrassing area of symptomology for men to talk about but it helps to be able to relate to other male patients going through the same things. I do have a moderate to good sex drive back now, since being on thyroid hormone replacement treatment that has been optimized for me by my current treating doctor.

The same is true of the emotions. They will improve with treatment over time but if you go through an especially bad time at some point, emotion-wise, don't hesitate to get extra help with that via medications or therapy if you have to. It's definitely not something to be ashamed of or embarrassed about because you certainly can't help the fact that you have a medical condition going on in your body!

Everything you described in your symptoms, I've been through and I can tell you with absolute assuredness that it will all improve over time with your treatment. Also be aware that your body may occasionally kick-in with some symptoms during this process because of medication-dose adjustments and possible antibody flares on occasion as well (thyroiditis flares). Antibodies are connected to symptoms because they cause inflammation and can flare with extra stress or extra hard physical activity. This aspect is not often mentioned by medical sources but is true non-the-less." End of Quote

The following famous men had/have thyroid disease (mostly the autoimmune type).

• President George Bush Senior

• Bobby Engram, NFL wide receiver with the Seattle Seahawks

• John F. Kennedy Jr. diagnosed (Graves' disease) in 1999

• Second Pres. of the U.S. John Adams, is believed to have suffered from Graves' Disease

• Rod Stewart (musician) ...

...

• Ben Crenshaw (Pro Golfer)

• Carl Lewis (10 Olympic Gold Medals Track & Field)

• Joe Piscopo (actor)

• Charles Marion Russell (cowboy artist)

• Roger Ebert (movie critic)

CHAPTER THREE

Famous Thyroid Disease Sufferers are Increasing Public Awareness

The people listed below (including George H.W. Bush who is also listed in the previous chapter) have brought more attention to thyroid disease, which according to some medical sources, is the most common endocrine-gland disorder, with approximately half of all cases remaining undiagnosed. Public awareness about symptoms and tests needed to diagnose thyroid disorders will help more people understand how to receive needed diagnoses and treatments.

Oprah Winfrey - In the year 2007, the worlds most famous and beloved talk show host, Oprah Winfrey, came forward with her story of thyroid disease diagnosis.

While she has not specifically stated that her case of hypothyroidism (under-active thyroid) is caused by "Hashimoto's thyroiditis" (autoimmune type), her description of symptoms she has experienced, point to this disease as being the cause of her thyroid disorder.

In an interview with CBS news, Oprah stated that she had gone through a period of feeling on edge and an inability to get a full night's sleep for weeks at a time, followed by extreme tiredness, rapid weight gain and the need to sleep more hours than required by a healthy person. These are the phases that patients with Hashimoto's thyroiditis commonly go through. While Oprah has not revealed her treatment regimen in-detail, she has stated that it has not yet required her to be administered drugs of any kind. The facts on Oprah's case may change at any time following the writing of this chapter.

Gail Devers - A female Olympic gold medal winner in track (also mentioned previously) and field in 1992 and 1996, Gail Devers was training for the next Olympic Games that would be held in the summer of 2000, when in 1998 she experienced the onset of hyperthyroid symptoms (overactive thyroid). She was noticing rapid weight-loss, dry skin, fatigue and muscle weakness that began to hinder her ability to continue her training. She also began to experience hair-loss and the emotional symptoms of anxiety and depression.

Upon having her blood tested, it was revealed that Gail was suffering from "Graves' disease," the autoimmune type of hyperthyroidism but the diagnosis was delayed and caused her to experience severe muscle-loss in her legs. Her thyroid gland was destroyed through a treatment called "Radioactive Iodine Ablation" and afterward she was placed on lifelong thyroid hormone replacement therapy. She has since regained her health and has been involved in acting as a spokesperson for thyroid disease organizations to help increase public awareness.

George H. W. Bush - The first President Bush, who served his term of office from 1989-1993 began to experience a heart arrhythmia called "atrial fibrillation," in 1991. He also noticed he was short of breath and experiencing spells of profuse sweating.

Upon checking into a hospital, he was diagnosed with Graves' disease and given Radioactive Iodine treatment to ablate (destroy) his thyroid gland and he was afterward placed on hormone replacement therapy via the synthetic thyroid hormone drug - Synthroid.

Coincidentally, President Bush's wife, First Lady Barbara Bush was also diagnosed with Graves' disease - hyperthyroidism as was their dog Millie. All of these members of the Bush family were successfully treated and were restored to an improved state of health. The Bush's dog - Millie passed away of natural causes in the year 1997.

CHAPTER FOUR

Oprah Winfrey's Diagnosis of Hypothyroidism

Over the past few years, Oprah Winfrey has been giving bits and pieces in regard to suffering from an illness related to her thyroid as mentioned in the previous chapter but more recently, she is revealing more about it. This is a great thing on her part because this will add public awareness to the subject of thyroid diseases.

The thyroid experts, including the AACE (American Association of Clinical Endocrinologists) have already expressed their belief that up to half of people who suffer thyroid diseases remain undiagnosed. This is due to both patients and Doctors, not having more awareness about thyroid disease symptoms and about the blood tests that easily diagnose thyroid hormone imbalances.

The AACE has estimated that approximately 27-million Americans suffer thyroid disease, which is a huge number and this makes people like Oprah Winfrey, that much more of an asset in helping to educate the public in regard to thyroid disorders.

I'm hoping she will have shows in the future that are dedicated to the subject.

Oprah has stated in talking about her thyroid disease, that she has experienced hyperthyroid symptoms (sped up metabolism), that caused her anxiety symptoms and inability to sleep well for weeks at a time, followed by hypothyroid symptoms (slowed metabolism) which began causing her severe, ongoing fatigue and the need to sleep a great deal more than normal.

An Endocrinologist in New York, Dr. Samara Ginzburg of the Albert Einstein College of Medicine, has been quoted in recent articles as expressing his belief that Oprah suffers from the thyroid disease called "Hashimoto's thyroiditis", also referred to as "Chronic Lymphocytic thyroiditis". This type of thyroid disease, is autoimmune caused, meaning it is caused buy an overactive immune system, that sends out killer cells called "antibodies", that attack and over time also destroy the thyroid gland.

Medical research still has not found the cause for autoimmune diseases but some theories include the idea that it could be caused by childhood viruses.

People commonly carry these in their bodies, once exposed to them, for their entire lives. The immune system in failing to eradicate these viruses will eventually turn on the natural tissues that contain them, including the thyroid gland.

I, the author of this article, suffer from Hashimoto's thyroiditis and I can relate to the symptom phases Oprah Winfrey has gone through. I too went through hyperthyroid symptoms, including severe anxiety and sleeplessness, before experiencing the onset of hypothyroid symptoms, which caused me severe fatigue, very dry skin, joint and muscle aches and depressed mood. I know how this disease can affect people who are experiencing it and I am proud to see such an admired and highly recognized individual such as Oprah Winfrey, coming forward with her own testimony about having thyroid disease. This may result in more Americans being tested and diagnosed, so that they too can be treated.

Improving Life for Thyroid Patients

CHAPTER FIVE

Thyroid Research Every Doctor Should Know

There is an article published by The Journal of Clinical Endocrinology & Metabolism, titled: *"In Search of the Impossible Dream? Thyroid Hormone Replacement Therapy That Treats All Symptoms in All Hypothyroid Patients"*

The article points out the fact that many patients who are on hormone replacement therapy for hypothyroidism, do not always experience significant symptom relief. The study also points out a variety of reasons for this problem of unsatisfactory results from thyroid medication used to treat hypothyroidism. It also points out the fact that some patients are treated with T-4 only thyroid medications, when some might benefit more from a combination T-4 and T-3 medication. It makes mention of the fact that some patients may be under-treated by their Doctors with their hypothyroid medications in general.

While it is a very interesting study, I feel some mention of the fact that if hypothyroidism has "thyroid autoimmunity" as its cause, the disease itself has potential to cause symptoms.

This can be true, apart from hormone levels also being a consideration. There are medical research studies out there that confirm this fact as well.

There is another medical research article titled; *"Chronic autoimmune thyroiditis and rheumatic manifestations."* (PubMed).

In this article from the National Institutes of Health/National Library of Medicine website, "rheumatic Manifestations" (joint & muscle pain) in relation to Hashimoto's thyroiditis (common cause of hypothyroidism) is addressed. Here we have a medical research article that attributes this symptom problem to the underlying autoimmune disease and not to hormone levels only.

In other words a treated hypothyroid patient can achieve a euthyroid state (normalized thyroid hormone levels) but can potentially still experience rheumatic symptoms from the underlying thyroid autoimmunity.

The important point this articles makes, is the fact that correcting hypothyroidism, in some patients, will not always resolve their joint and muscle aches completely.

Doctors who believe their treated hypothyroid patients are imagining (psychosomatic) their unrelieved rheumatic symptoms, need to read this article.

Another article I wish to refer to is titled; *"A case control study on psychiatric disorders in Hashimoto disease and euthyroid goiter: not only depressive but also anxiety disorders are associated with thyroid autoimmunity"*

This article points out that Hashimoto's thyroiditis or the type of thyroid autoimmunity that causes hypothyroidism has the potential to cause "anxiety disorders" in addition to depression. They distinguish between hormone levels and the disease itself as a cause of emotional disorders. Some Doctors tell patients their emotional symptoms are not related to their thyroid disease but these type research articles say differently. A number of other research articles confirm this same conclusion.

The next research article I wish to refer to, is titled; *"Association between thyroid autoimmunity and fibromyalgic disease severity"* (Journal Clinical Rheumatology)

In this article found in the Journal of Clinical Rheumatology, an association between thyroid autoimmunity and fibromyalgia is noted. This is only one of many research articles that connect thyroid disease to fibromyalgia. Other articles make a connection specifically of "TPO antibodies" (one of the antibodies that causes Hashimoto's thyroiditis) to fibromyalgia and that people with fibromyalgia commonly have sub-clinical hypothyroidism, rather than full blown or overt hypothyroidism. There are many more research articles in addition to this one that connects thyroid disease to fibromyalgia.

The next article I wish to point out is titled; *"Modifications of the Immune Responsiveness in Patients with Autoimmune Thyroiditis: Evidence for a Systemic Immune Alteration".*

This research article concludes that a degree of "peripheral immune deficiency" is present in patients with "Hashimoto's thyroiditis", the most common cause of hypothyroidism. The importance of this article in my opinion is in recognizing that autoimmune hypothyroid disease has a "systemic" (system-wide) effect on these patient's immune systems.

This may help explain why patients with thyroid autoimmunity have a higher susceptibility for developing other autoimmune diseases and health disorders of many kinds. It also can help to explain why all symptoms are not relieved in all patients on hormone therapy for autoimmune hypothyroidism because correction of the hypothyroidism may not necessarily mean correction of the disease affecting the immune system as a whole.

Here's an interesting one I wish to point out as well, titled *"Fibromyalgia and Thyroid Function"* (Genova Diagnostics)

In this article published by "GDX", in regard to the association between thyroid dysfunction and fibromyalgia, the article cites other studies and mentions the statistics from studies that report that up to 80% of fibromyalgia patients may suffer from some form of sub clinical hypothyroidism.

This last medical research article I wish to refer to is titled; *"Assessment of Anxiety in Sub-clinical Thyroid Disorders"* (Science Links Japan)

This article was published in an Endocrine Journal in Japan and also added to the links on the Science Links Japan website and is on the subject of "anxiety" as it manifests in sub-clinical thyroid disorders. The conclusion in this medical study is that anxiety can develop in sub-clinical thyroid disorders whether hyperthyroid or hypothyroid. This lends toward correcting the misperception by some in the medical community who believe only hyperthyroid states cause anxiety symptoms. It is also in opposition to some opinions that state only full blown thyroid dysfunction causes emotional symptoms. This article points out that patients with sub-clinical thyroid dysfunction can potentially experience anxiety symptoms.

CHAPTER SIX

Thyroid Hormone Replacement and Antidepressants

I have discussed this subject often in articles and on forums but I want to say, as I always do, that antidepressants are greatly helpful to many people and in fact have probably been lifesavers for many as well.

One disease that commonly causes anxiety and depression as part of the symptoms is thyroid disease that results in hyperthyroidism (over-active) or hypothyroidism (under-active) plus there are other many other diseases and health disorders that cause emotional symptoms as well.

I believe if a thyroid patient is on adequate treatment/hormone therapy but still needs the added help of antidepressant, there is nothing at all wrong with this. Having said this, let me now point out problems I see with Doctors who do not first give thyroid hormone replacement time to work, before adding an antidepressant to a patient's treatment. Certainly Thyroid HRT (thyroid hormone therapy) has the potential to relieve symptoms greatly.

I'll say in my case, the emotional symptoms of anxiety and depression were some of the first ones helped the most, when I was treated and this alone was a great accomplishment.

What was not good in my case and that of many other patients I have corresponded with or whose stories I have read is that I was originally "diagnosed" with emotional-only problems and the thyroid disease was not blood-tested for. Because of this, my fatigue, joint pain, dry skin, etc...., did not improve on the antidepressant alone but actually worsened. This combined with the side effects, caused me to slowly wean off the SSRI antidepressant (this should always be done with Dr.-supervision) and in the mean time, blood tests I demanded and had blood drawn for, just prior to starting the mood drug, revealed thyroid disease, including hypothyroidism and highly elevated thyroid antibody levels.

The problem I saw in my GP pushing constantly for me to resume the antidepressant, along with my thyroid medication, was that there was the potential for me to confuse the SSRI side-effects, with unrelieved thyroid symptoms.

The side-effects after all, include some of those that are identical to hypothyroidism/thyroid disease; "fatigue, tremor, nervousness, lightheadedness etc..."

In my opinion, thyroid disease symptoms, including depression/anxiety, should be monitored with hormone treatment, to see how much they improve and if they do not begin improving after a few weeks, an SSRI and other medications, such as those for muscle/joint aches etc..., can be added. I believe if anxiety and/or depression is thyroid disease related, obviously hormone replacement therapy has even more potential to improve it, than an antidepressant does.

Another problem is "withdrawal". Patients, who have been on an antidepressant, will experience a worsening of the emotional symptoms, plus other withdrawal symptoms, when coming off an antidepressant and they will mistakenly believe this means the emotional symptoms are severe without the SSRI, when in reality; this is a common reaction when tapering off of one.

If a patient, with Dr. Supervision, decides to taper off an antidepressant, it must be done very slowly, with withdrawal symptoms monitored closely.

Some patients actually have become suicidal from withdrawal, while others don't have as difficult a time.

If a patient does not have a problem with the possibility of needing antidepressants as lifelong treatment and they do indeed need the drug (and many do), then they should make the decision to remain on them as long as is necessary but if at some point they want to wean off of the drug, it should be done slowly and very cautiously and never without the supervision of a qualified Doctor.

While antidepressant medications are very helpful and necessary under the right conditions, consideration should also be given to the possibility of underlying medical causes of emotional symptoms that must also be diagnosed and treated, with adequate time for disease-treatment to resolve symptoms.

CHAPTER SEVEN

Stress Management for Thyroid Patients

According to the PubMed published medical research article titled; *"STRESS AND THYROID AUTOIMMUNITY"*, stress plays a role in triggering the onset of autoimmune thyroid diseases.

Quote: "Stress can be one of the environmental factors for thyroid autoimmunity."

One skill that few people truly possess would have to be successful stress management. Stress seems to play a major role in most of our daily lives but we can benefit greatly from mastering or at least improving the skill of stress management. There are so many ways that stress affects our lives, even in ways that we might not recognize. There are many effective ways to manage stress levels so that you can begin living a life that is less harmful to your mind, emotions and body.

Stress can continually be a major problem in a person's life especially in these days of living in this crazy, hectic, fast-paced world.

Stress can be brought on and aggravated by many things both major and minor including work, personal life problems, financial issues, relationships, school, children, health problems, or many times from an overload of all these things combined. Some people even become stressed over the little things such as traffic, a long line at the grocery store, house chores and upcoming events or even because a waiter treated you badly at a restaurant. These are just a few examples but there are many things that cause stress in people's lives that can accumulate and become harmful over time.

There are many stress-relievers available for practice to help us deal with the "stressors" of daily life. Yoga and meditation are very popular ways that can help us experience some relief from the stressors of a hectic life. Exercise in general is also a great way to deal with excessive stress. Having an occasional quiet time can also provide some stress reduction, by removing ourselves from everything and everyone for a few minutes a day. This can help us to calm down and place us back into focus.

Deep breathing exercises are another good way to relieve stress, by taking, slow, long, deep breaths, inflating your diaphragm, rather than your chest.

Some people suffer stress that is severe enough that they need the help of a therapist or a medication to deal with it. This can actually be a good idea if you are suffering stress severe enough, that you are losing the ability to handle it well on your own. Hobbies and leisure activities that you enjoy can also be stress relievers. Activities involving art projects, such as painting, drawing, building things, scrap-booking, and gardening are a few simple ways to get your mind off of all the stressors you are experiencing and to enjoy some leisure time.

The consequences of not mastering the skill of stress management may include health problems, depression, and lack of sleep to name a few. Stress can contribute to or even be a cause of these health issues that can be potentially harmful if stress is not brought under control. Other health problems may also include muscle tension, increased heart rate, headaches, increased blood pressure (hypertension), increased risk for heart attack and stroke.

It can also cause more vulnerability to colds, viruses and may also increase the risk for developing certain types of diseases. Stress can also take away much the happiness in life and cause symptoms of anxiety and cause increased susceptibility to depression. For these reasons it is very important to work on these skills for mastering stress.

Another way in helping to master stress management is to identify all of the things that stress you out and to begin working on improving these areas. A simple method for helping to identify stressors is to write it down in a notebook each time you find yourself getting stressed about something. This will help you identify those stressors, so that you can begin to work on ways to better deal with, reduce them and possibly even eliminate them. Also, try working on ways to stop any negative thought patterns that contribute to stress as soon as they begin coming into your mind. Try to think positively no matter what the situation might be because it is very likely that your concerns are not as bad as you have allowed yourself to think they are.

You have to develop a practice of controlling your negative responses to stressful thoughts and learn to better cope with them.

Also try to remove yourself from any situations that cause added stress for you, whether it is certain job situations or even a relationship that causes ongoing stress.

If you can identify anything that is negatively affecting your daily life, it is important to remove yourself from those things if at all possible, since they will only serve to make your life more difficult and complicated than it should reasonably have to be.

Most people can benefit in many ways from mastering these skills for reducing stress which can lend toward a much happier and healthier life.

The benefits of better health that can result are not only physical but also mental and emotional. Mastering these skills can also help you to benefit more from life itself and help you to experience more enjoyment in life as well.

Hopefully more people will begin to realize that chronic stress is a continually growing problem in our society and causes an increase in negative and violent behaviors. We all must begin working more on skills and methods for coping because stress can easily spiral out of control if we do not do everything we can to control it instead of allowing it to control us.

CHAPTER EIGHT

Anxiety and Depression in Thyroid Disease

In the year 2002, I was experiencing the onset of hypothyroidism from Hashimoto's Disease and some of the more concerning symptoms I had were the emotional ones as mentioned previously. Once I was diagnosed and began treatment, these symptoms improved dramatically. As all of this was happening; I began to research intensely, finding out all I could about every aspect of thyroid disease and the symptoms, plus co-existing disorders that can also manifest in persons with thyroid diseases. I would like to share some of those things I learned.

According to many reputable, quality medical resources I studied on, about thyroid disease and its symptoms, I learned that in many people, the emotional symptoms are the first ones that are experienced. Many times, subtle symptoms of depression and anxiety begin to be experienced and over time these will worsen if the patient doesn't receive treatment.

Doctors will often first think a patient is experiencing emotional problems only and will prescribe patients, antidepressants. Of course the person with thyroid disease is experiencing emotional problems but the root cause is thyroid disease and so treatment is needed before the emotional symptoms will have any significant improvement.

There is nothing wrong with patients needing antidepressant medications as mentioned previously but in the case of a thyroid patient, an antidepressant alone will not resolve the root-problem. On the other hand, some thyroid patients take antidepressants and other medications to help with emotional symptoms, while also being treated for their thyroid disease and there is certainly nothing wrong with this either as long as the medical condition is getting the attention that is needed.

Many of the medical research articles I have read, also state that the emotional symptoms of autoimmune thyroid diseases (the most common type), are not only the result of the abnormal thyroid hormone levels but also from the actual autoimmune disease process itself.

Improving Life for Thyroid Patients

Anti-Thyroid antibodies such as the TPO (anti-thyroid-peroxidase) and TG (anti-thyroglobulin) ones, when elevated, can contribute to anxiety and depression symptoms, even before thyroid hormone levels become abnormal. Many of these studies concluded that patients with positive thyroid antibodies, may also experience joint pain and fibromyalgia type symptoms from the elevated antibody levels.

People, who experience the onset of emotional symptoms, should have thorough examination by their doctor and a thorough blood lab work-up, to determine if the cause is a medical condition such as thyroid disease. If it is found to be the case, treatment for thyroid hormone imbalance can help significantly with symptoms of anxiety and/or depression.

Thyroid Disease Support Groups

Thyroid patients often relate better to fellow-patients who are going through similar struggles to find effective treatments, symptom relief and best quality-of-life. Many patients who have corresponded with me over the years, asked for my advice regarding coping emotionally with their disease.

I have often referred them to patient support groups. Following below, I will also offer advice on starting a support group in your area if one is not already available.

Fellow-patient thyroid disease support groups can offer the opportunity for patients to meet and share advice and personal experiences. The benefits of regular meetings in-person or online can also provide opportunity for helpful, reliable resources to be shared among patients who can refer one another to informative books and helpful online information they have found. Meetings can also open discussions on important thyroid topics members may wish to participate-in to help them gain general knowledge about their disease and its treatment.

Publicly Announcing a New Support Group

One effective way to inform the public in one's own area about the formation of a new thyroid disease support group is to submit an announcement covering the event in a local newspaper. Local media is often helpful with offering free coverage for something that will be helpful to their community.

Written coverage for the support group might be submitted as a letter to the editor, for inclusion in that section or as a news story or press release that contains information in regard to the importance for thyroid patients in the area for such a resource to become available.

The announcement submitter might also consider relating a brief personal story within the submission to the newspaper that demonstrates the need patients have in connecting to other patients and to sources of shared information that can help them cope with their disease emotionally. If a newspaper is reluctant to allow free coverage of the event, a paid advertisement might be a consideration. Local radio stations may also agree to inform the public at no charge by airing announcements for the support group. Typing up fliers on a computer and printing them for distribution to bulletin boards and for handing out can also help get the word out.

Support Group Newsletter

The support group director or those appointed to plan meetings may also consider publishing a monthly or bi-monthly newsletter to inform members about times set for meetings.

It can also provide an outline of the information that will be covered in them. The newsletter publisher might also offer opportunity for members to submit personal stories and/or helpful information from reliable, reputable sources, for consideration of being added into the newsletter. It can also be offered to the local public in-general whether they decide to become eventual members or not. Personal stories, book reviews and covering discussions taking place in meetings can help gain more interest for the support group. A newsletter can be offered through email and/or in print.

Inviting Guest Speakers

Special guests can be invited to make presentations or to give lectures on thyroid disease subjects for the support group. Area doctors that treat thyroid diseases might be interested in making guest appearances to relate helpful information to thyroid patient members. Subjects of interest covered by guest speakers might include those pertaining to the diet practices of thyroid patients, partnering with their doctors, best methods for taking their medications and any other subject of interest for the group, to help better inform them.

Improving Life for Thyroid Patients

Providing an Online Forum

A support group administrator might also choose to create an accompanying forum for members who may wish to communicate between meetings or might actually choose to create the support group as a whole, as an online resource. A forum requires a degree of moderation, so that unwanted posts or spam can be deleted or edited. The forum could also be restricted to those who are members of the support group. A forum can be a great resource of ongoing communication, for added support and shared information.

The forum moderator(s) would also want to put effort into making sure the forum stays on-subject for each topic-category that might be included in the forum and to make sure small offshoots of members are not formed which can sometimes evolve into exclusionary cliques. Any hurtful practices would also need to be addressed such as gossip or posts that degrade into personal attacks. If these types of things are closely moderated, a forum can be an excellent resource for thyroid disease patients and some online hosts make forums available free of charge.

Online Thyroid Support and Information

The internet contains a wonderful source of helpful information and places of emotional support offered to patients suffering chronic diseases, including thyroid-related ones. Patients suffering under-active and overactive thyroid disorder symptoms can connect to fellow patients and become self-educated about the disease that is affecting their lives.

Thyroid Patient Advocate Information Sites

There are a large number of dependable and reputable information sources online that supply helpful information that can be relied upon, on a full range of thyroid related subjects. You'll find articles on hyperthyroid, hypothyroid, and thyroid autoimmunity conditions and about symptom manifestations that are experienced with these disorders.

Many of the writers of online thyroid disease information are also fellow thyroid patients or what are also referred to as "Thyroid Patient Advocates".

There are website information sources by well-studied patient advocates who are also well recognized authors of best selling books on thyroid subjects, including Elaine Moore of Suite101.com and Mary Shomon, creator of the thyroid-info.com website. Patients can take advantage of the great information offered by these authors, both online and by obtaining their books in print.

Medical Thyroid Information Sites

These type sites offer information from a purely medical standpoint, without the fellow-patient view but can also be greatly instrumental in helping thyroid patients become better educated about their disorders. While doctors can help patients gain a general understanding about their conditions, they seldom have the time needed to fully educate their patients as they desire to be. Learning about a disease that is often life-long and that can cause a degree of change in activity and lifestyle by patients who suffer them, can help take away some of the fear and uncertainty from the experience, especially in newly diagnosed patients.

Medical thyroid information sites that can be helpful to patients include the American Thyroid Association, Thyroid Disease Manager and the American Thyroid Association (patient brochures).

Patient Blogs and Forums

Many patients have blogs online, on which they post ongoing information about their personal experience with thyroid disease, including their emotional struggles. Other patients reading their posts can find experiences they relate to, that can help them feel less-alone with their disease. Some blogs also allow posting via message boards or forums that are available on their pages. Other forums and message boards are for the sole purpose of posting thyroid-related questions and for fellow-patient information sharing and support. Some are also moderated by volunteer medical professionals who reply to patient's questions.

An online search using Google or other search engines, including the keywords "thyroid blogs", "personal thyroid stories" and "thyroid forums and message boards", will yield many pages showing the available resources in these areas.

Improving Life for Thyroid Patients

Thyroid patients who feel the need for emotional support and/or information can take advantage of these type resources and if they do not own a computer, can go online free of charge at a public library.

CHAPTER NINE

My Experience with Thyroid Related Anxiety and Panic

As I began developing hypothyroidism from autoimmune thyroid disease (Hashimoto's), I began having serious anxiety attacks and panic attacks. Many patients experience these, just as the thyroid gland begins to fail and become hypothyroid as addressed in previous chapters. With Grave's Disease patients (Autoimmune-Hyperthyroidism), they too will have the anxiety symptoms but they are many times experienced continuously, until they can begin treatment to slow down the overproduction of their thyroid glands.

My anxiety was intermittent and would alternate with spells of depression. Researchers describe the anxiety symptoms from autoimmune hypothyroidism, as sometimes being caused by the gland's attempt to "sputter back to life" as it begins to fail in attempt to fight off the autoimmune attack. The actual medical term for this is "Hashitoxicosis" and patients will have it to varying degrees but usually it is a milder form that can still causes significant anxiety symptoms.

48

Following are some of the more common symptoms of anxiety that can be experienced.

• sudden intense feelings of fear

• rapid heart rate

• elevated blood pressure

• rapid breathing (hyperventilation)

• sweating, trembling

• muscle tension with pain (including chest area)

There can also be anxiety that is more of a constant type keyed-up feeling, called "free floating anxiety" that causes a continuous nervous feeling of being on-edge that thyroid patients can experience.

This also brings on feelings of constant, chronic worry that is referred to as "Generalized Anxiety Disorder". The more intense episodes of anxiety come under the heading of "anxiety attacks" and "panic attacks". These obviously are very unpleasant and there were times I personally would experience these, during the night, causing me to awaken in a cold sweat, while also experiencing the other described symptoms.

Improving Life for Thyroid Patients

There are also the symptoms of depression that are common to thyroid disease patients, especially prior to being treated. The more common ones include following.

• feeling slowed down

• inability to enjoy things

• sadness

• irritability

• anger

• feelings of hopelessness (sometimes including suicidal thoughts)

• feeling tired and lethargic

The symptoms of depression can co-exist with anxiety or sometimes will alternate so that a thyroid patient experiences anxiety part of the time and depression the other part of the time.

My own emotional symptoms were some of the first to resolve with thyroid hormone replacement therapy.

I still have occasional mild flares of anxiety and depression symptoms due to having the autoimmune thyroid disease but the improvements over my pre-treatment state have been significant.

Thyroid patients suffering emotional symptoms should be encouraged to know that hormone replacement therapy can potentially improve these symptoms significantly. If it does not do so adequately in some patients, there are medication options out there that are effective in treating emotional symptoms.

With Hashimoto's, you can go through a period of "Hashitoxicosis" (actual medical term) as mentioned earlier, especially early into the onset of hypothyroidism which causes thyroid to waiver back and forth between producing low hormone and having surges of increased hormone, as it tries to avoid hypothyroidism and intermittently spurts back to life. This is a real condition and I've seen the testimonies of literally 100s of patients that experience panic attacks from it and I am one who experienced them for a time when I was newly diagnosed. Some medical sources state that Hashitoxicosis is rare, while I personally believe it is common in milder forms.

Strangely some doctors do not seem to know about this condition that goes with autoimmune hypothyroidism. They will actually tell patients their anxiety is not caused by the diagnosed thyroid disease but is a separate issue and many times they will prescribe additional medications for it, before giving thyroid hormone medication a chance to work.

There is a Dr. Richard Hall MD, also a professor of psychiatry, who has been involved in research studies at major medical universities, such as John Hopkins University and in his studies on the relationship of anxiety to endocrine disorders it was found that in patients with "Hashimoto's thyroiditis", anxiety was a common, prominent symptom at the time patients were diagnosed.

There are also studies that have been published on the "PubMed" website, which is provided by the U.S. National Institutes of Health and the National Library of Medicine, stating that anxiety symptoms and anxiety disorders are associated with Hashimoto's disease, which is also the most common cause of hypothyroidism in industrialized countries.

It is important that your diagnosed thyroid disease be treated optimally because some Doctors believe simply getting your TSH and thyroid hormone levels anywhere into the normal range is adequate treatment with thyroid hormone replacement medication (TSH elevates with hypothyroidism and thyroid hormones decrease). The truth is however that, your better Endocrinologists and Thyroid Specialists have a more targeted therapeutic treatment goal (the average TSH normal values is "0.5 to 5.0"). They will for example have a TSH treatment goal of suppressing it down to a "1.0" target range. Depending on a patient's symptoms, they might even get it down to the lower normal TSH range of from 0.3 to 0.5, to see if a patient has better resolution of symptoms.

These are just some points I thought I would share because over time, adequate treatment will help a great deal in resolving anxiety and other symptoms of autoimmune hypothyroidism. Thyroid hormone replacement medication serves to take over and supply thyroid hormone to the body, while causing a person's own thyroid gland to be suppressed (TSH suppression).

A patient then begins to see more properly leveled-out thyroid hormones in the body, rather than the erratic changes in levels, a dying thyroid produces before treatment takes over.

In the mean time as a patient waits for symptom improvements, help with medication for anxiety, is nothing to be ashamed of or afraid of, if needed while thyroid treatment is being optimized, which can actually take several months in some cases. Some medical sources suggest that thyroid hormone replacement therapy for hypothyroidism, takes only 4 to 6 weeks to do its job but this simply is not true with a large percent of patients, who may need several dosage adjustments over several months, before they reach their optimal treatment level.

If you are taking an antidepressant and it is not working as it should (these are also prescribed for anxiety) or it is causing unwanted side effects, you might discuss with your Doctor, slowly weaning off of it and being place on a trial of an "as-needed" anti-anxiety medication, that can be taken short-term, rather than the type that must be built-up in your system and maintained as a permanent daily regimen.

Some patients do fine with the permanent antidepressant type drugs, while others may not.

Some Doctors seem to believe SSRI and other types of antidepressants work well for everyone they are prescribed to but this simply is not true in some cases. I have corresponded with dozens of thyroid patients, who simply could not adjust well to them even after several months of trying to benefit, while many others do very well on them. People are individuals and nothing works exactly the same for everyone and is a common sense approach that Doctors should take with these type drugs.

CHAPTER TEN

More of My Personal Thyroid Story

I have suffered several disorders/diseases during my lifetime, the most recent and the one most profoundly affecting me, being Hashimoto's Disease/Hypothyroidism.

My first experience with a disorder causing me symptoms was in my teen years, during the 1970s, being diagnosed with what an MD and Cardiologist thought was "Wolf-Parkinson-White Syndrome", due to finding a "click-murmur" but turns out I was experiencing Mitral Valve Prolapse Syndrome for all those years. The condition has at times caused me panic attacks and generalized anxiety, spells of tachycardia, orthostatic hypotension/dysautonomia (dizziness upon first standing up), fatigue, exercise intolerance etc...

Now fast forward to the year 2001. I went back to a heart specialist at age-38 and he ruled-out my ever having Wolf-Parkinson-White Syndrome and said I could not have previously had the murmur, being a condition that is lifelong unless corrected by surgery.

A couple of years later, through online research, I found information on Mitral Valve Prolapse Syndrome (symptoms from MVP) and realized this is what these doctors were detecting.

Unless a Dr. specifically tests for Mitral Valve Prolapse, most of the time, they will not find it incidentally because it is a common heart murmur (statistics: affects 5% to 20% of the population) and they don't give the condition a great deal of credence unless a patient experiences symptoms ("MVP-Syndrome"). My mother has had the same symptoms as mine for most of her life and was diagnosed with MVP and mild co-morbid regurgitation (mild blood seepage from the valve), plus both my son and daughter have the MVP symptoms (the murmur runs in families). My daughter also has "Pectus-Excavatum", a curvature of the spine that commonly co-exists with MVP.

I was very pleased that the Cardiologist, ruled out the more serious type heart murmur but following this revelation of having MVP instead, I began developing new, more severe symptoms. I also broke out in a severe case of hives, which I had never experienced before in my life.

A Doctor prescribed antihistamines and I recovered from the hives but I had worsening onset of fatigue, dry skin, more hair falling out, anxiety/depression, constipation and joint pain.

I made a new Doctor visit and even though I actually suggested the possibility of thyroid problems, the Doctor prescribed me antidepressants. As I took these for only a few weeks, my symptoms worsened because the underlying thyroid disease wasn't being diagnosed and treated.

Before starting the antidepressant, I called a new Doctor and asked for a blood draw so that thyroid tests could be done in addition to a CBC and a fasting glucose level. My TSH, the pituitary hormone that reflects the thyroid hormone levels was in a range of "0.35 to 4.5" and was flagged high at "8.3" (increased due to hypothyroidism). I also had a T-3 Uptake flagged two percents below normal and all my actual thyroid hormone levels (T4 and T3) were in the lower half of normal. The Doctor almost didn't agree to start treating me, being one from the camp that believes TSH must be above a "10" for treatment to be considered but he agreed to place me on low-dose Synthroid (synthetic T4 replacement) due to my symptoms.

58

I changed Doctors again after a few months of experiencing a lack of improvement and was placed on a higher dose of Synthroid, later changed to "Armour thyroid" brand, when symptoms didn't improve. My Doctor at that time thought my lack of improvement was due to "inadequate conversion" by my body, of T-4, into T-3 (the latter being more metabolically active) but in reality, I was not on a high enough dose of T4-only thyroid hormone replacement medication, to make me feel well. I did extensive researching and found that the dose I was on for the first two years of my treatment was inadequate – I was being under treated.

The Doctor who first treated me only had my TSH suppressed down to "4.95" and because of a different lab he used, having a TSH range of "0.5 to 5.0", he said that this was a "perfect" reading. I wondered why I was still feeling sick, so was having other testing done and in the process, I had a 24-hour urine cortisol and 10 different saliva cortisol tests that revealed I was also experiencing "adrenal fatigue" (sub clinical adrenal insufficiency) and because of this, my thyroid medication was not adjusting in my body properly.

After a few months on replacement thyroid hormones, I developed increased joint pain, fatigue, swollen lymph glands and severe post exertional malaise (fatigue following mild exertion).

My newest Doctor's response to my urine-cortisol being very low-normal and four different saliva cortisol tests being flagged clinically low and others never being above lowest-normal, was that I had a hypo-functioning "HPA Axis" (Hypothalamous-Pituitary-Adrenals) and that there was treatment for it. I immediately began researching online again and found that I was experiencing "Chronic Fatigue Syndrome", triggered by a combination of Hashimoto's Hypothyroidism, vitamin deficiencies and Adrenal Fatigue. What I needed was to support my adrenals and treat my low vitamin levels, along with increasing my thyroid medication, to recover from this terrible syndrome!

I found yet another Endocrinologist, who placed me on a higher dose of Armour, one that brought my TSH down to between a 1.0 and 0.3 and I felt better almost immediately.

Also, since none of the previous Doctors checked my TPO and TG Thyroid Antibodies, to see if the cause of my hypothyroidism was "thyroid autoimmunity" I had these checked after two years on thyroid hormone medication. My TG ABs, were highly elevated @ "537" (range <40) and my TPO ABs were @ "84" (range <35). This revealed the Hashimoto's thyroiditis.

More Doctors are recognizing the need to treat patients individually, rather than thinking we all fit into the same mold. More of them are also realizing that a normal TSH range is not normal for everyone. The AACE recognized this several years ago, when they revised the old TSH range to "0.3 to 3.0", from the old one that was generally in the "0.5 to 5.0" range. Also, the "diagnostic range", is not the same as the "treatment range" for TSH.

Doctors who have published articles with the AACE suggest that patients on thyroid hormone medication, should have a TSH between "1.0 to 2.0", however, I have corresponded with several Board Certified Endocrinologists, who have stated that many patients need to have their treatment-goal TSH to be between "0.3 to 1.0".

This level is sometimes needed to successfully relieve hypothyroidism symptoms and a few patients may need even lower-normal TSH levels as previously mentioned. These types of patients of course must be monitored closely.

As I was administered the higher thyroid medication dose, I also began taking vitamin supplements, containing those needed to boost my adrenals and fix my deficiencies, plus I was taking some low-dose adrenal glandular (beef source) and low-dose DHEA (over-the-counter androgen hormone), for relatively short term. The combination of higher thyroid dose and boosting my adrenals, gave me wonderful improvement that I had not experienced previously. I have maintained this improvement for several years now. I still have days of not feeling quit 100% but I feel some thyroid patients will have fluctuations of symptoms, due to the autoimmune process itself, while others may not.

CHAPTER ELEVEN

Treated Hypothyroidism and Weight Gain

It is a well known fact that untreated hypothyroidism causes moderate weight gain, in fact some patients report weight gain that is in excess of moderate. I use the term moderate however, because most medical sources state it as such and they also suggest that weight gain with untreated hypothyroidism will usually not result in more than 20lb of weight gain.

Regardless of the actual amount of weight gain, which in my opinion varies among individual patients and depends upon how severe their untreated hypothyroidism is, it does indeed cause weight gain!

This is due to the fact that with hypothyroid conditions, the rate of our bodily metabolism is slowed down. We burn less energy when the metabolism is not running at a normal rate. They also refer to this as hypo-metabolism, which can have additional causes other than hypothyroidism.

When we look at patients who are being treated for hypothyroidism whether from hypothyroid disease or following treatment for hyperthyroidism (i.e. thyroid removal), we still hear them report gaining weight more easily and having difficulty losing weight. There are no medical research studies on the subject of weight gain in patients being treated for hypothyroidism that I am aware of but the number of patients attesting to this problem in online articles and on patient forums is significant. I personally can also attest to the fact that I too gain weight more easily and have a harder time losing weight, despite being adequately and even optimally treated for my hypothyroidism.

I'm not sure we will ever have a firm medical explanation as to why this happens but it could possibly be that thyroid hormone being administered from the outside (hormone therapy), whether it is the natural or synthetic form, is slightly less effective in regulating bodily metabolism than naturally occurring human hormone is. This is certainly just a theory but in my opinion, is a reasonable one that should be given some consideration by those in the medical profession.

Another theory that I believe should be considered, is the possibility that "thyroid autoimmunity" that is present in most cases of hypothyroidism, may also play a factor in weight control. It may be that thyroid antibodies also affect our metabolism, to a very small degree but significant enough to affect our body's ability to burn calories and to turn fat into energy. I do know that "insulin resistance" is more common in treated hypothyroid patients and the description I just gave, fits this condition. I can also attest to being a hypothyroid patient with co-morbid insulin resistance.

Treated hypothyroid patients must work harder than people without thyroid disease, to lose weight and to keep their weight under control. While there are many diet plans out there, I feel the same principles apply in weight loss, no matter which diet plan you may try. The principles include eating healthier, which would consist of eating more fruits, vegetables, nuts and grains, cutting back and eliminating refined sugars from your diet, eating less and exercising more.

These principles can be wrapped together in many different packages and called by many different diet-plan names but they are the principles that work and you simply add discipline to that plan, to make it successful.

Weight gain and difficulty losing weight is a challenge to treated hypothyroid patients but one they can accomplish with effort.

CHAPTER TWELVE

Book Review for "Hypothyroidism Type 2"

As a Thyroid Patient Advocate, I am inspired to direct fellow-patients and others interested in thyroid disease subjects, to other resources that have important educational value. In this chapter I wish to add a review of a book I feel is very important in the area of symptoms and diagnosis of a variant of hypothyroidism that the book's author has named "Hypothyroidism Type 2". It is my belief that more public awareness of this growing problem in regard to under-active thyroid cases that are subtle in manifestation is very important. This book is highly instrumental in helping to accomplish this and I highly recommend it as an information resource on thyroid disease.

Doctor Mark Starr brings to light, hypothyroid conditions that are genetic and due to inherited problems with thyroid hormone metabolism and environmental toxins in this book titled; "Hypothyroidism Type 2".

Can hypothyroidism in some people be undetectable by blood testing or imaging tests alone? Medical evidence going back many years would seem to confirm this to be the case. There are in fact subtle but chronic cases of low-grade hypothyroidism that blood labs do not detect and yet the signs and symptoms for hypothyroidism are present. In cases when this type hypothyroidism is suspected, other testing methods may need to be undertaken to confirm or rule-out the presence of Hypothyroidism Type 2. (Special thanks, to Dr. Starr for a free review copy of the book.)

Hypothyroidism Diagnoses Prior to Blood Testing

Doctor Starr's book covers an array of fascinating aspects in regard to both the early years and present-day methods for diagnosing hypothyroidism. The major diagnosing method for hypothyroidism before the advent of blood labs for thyroid evaluation was observing patients for "myxedema", meaning that a patient had marked puffiness from swelling in tissues of the body.

In fact the term myxedema was an early one describing hypothyroidism in-general and the two terms were used interchangeably for many years following.

Methods for measuring a patient's metabolism were also used in the early days, including a measure of how much oxygen a patient was using within a determined period of time, with lower than normal usage indicating a slowed metabolism. The metabolic body temperatures of people suspected of having hypothyroidism were also measured, which is referred to as the "basal body temperature", a below-normal reading indicating hypothyroidism. The book points out the fact that cases of elusive hypothyroidism may require diagnosing via these early methods, which may actually be more reliable in detecting subtle cases.

Doctor Starr's Credentials

Studying the research of endocrinology pioneers, Dr. Starr, who is Board Certified in Pain Medicine, has dedicated decades of study to research by W.M. Ord, a British researcher who discovered autoimmune thyroiditis in 1877 and who is also responsible for the term "myxedema".

He has also extensively studied the research of Dr. Broda O. Barnes who developed the early testing methods of oxygen-use measuring and basal body temperature methods for detecting hypothyroidism. Additionally, he studied directly with the late Professor Hans Kraus, formerly of the Rusk Institute and the MD who also treated John F. Kennedy's Addison's disease and hypothyroidism in the early 1960s.

Not only did Dr. Starr discover his own Hypothyroidism Type 2 but also diagnosed and treated Dr. Thomas D. Broc, B.Sc., D.D.S., whom also suffered hypothyroidism that was elusive to blood testing. A foreword by Dr. Broc is included in the book that expresses deep appreciation to Dr. Starr whose treatment with thyroid hormone replacement was instrumental in resolving a pain syndrome being experienced by Dr. Broc.

Other Aspects Covered In the Book

Dr. Starr dedicates pages in this book, to the subject of "mitochondria" (cells that produce energy in the body) and how these very important cells are sometimes hindered in this function by environmental pollutants and toxins and by faulty genes inherited by predisposed individuals.

The studies cited in these areas and the documentation provided, is impressive and includes those involving autopsy studies and umbilical cord studies which have strongly confirmed the effects of environmental toxins on mitochondria and thyroid hormone metabolism.

Are there controversial areas of research covered in the book? There certainly are and Dr. Starr is aware of this but despite this, facts contained in the book are fully documented by a great deal of medical research and is an extremely interesting read for both doctors and laypersons with interest in thyroid disease subjects.

CHAPTER THIRTEEN

Embracing Your Thyroid Disease?

Once seeing the title of this chapter, you may be questioning what in the world does it mean to "embrace and accept your thyroid disease" and what would it mean to embrace or accept any disease for that matter?

Certainly I am not of the belief that we should be accepting of a disease that might invade our bodies and become a part of us or that we should appreciate a disease for doing so. What I'm saying is that once we have experienced the onset of a disease and have been diagnosed, we should reserve ourselves to the fact that the disease has indeed become a part of us, at least for the time being.

It is very important that we find positive avenues for dealing with the illness, otherwise, we will find ourselves in a tremendous struggle and negative battle against something that at least for the time being, we do not have complete control of.

I once heard an Osteopath doctor, who is also a Christian, tell a patient not to anguish about their disease, which was a form of cancer and potentially life-threatening. He told this patient that for the time-being, it was better to simply go with the flow and not battle against the disease with constant worry or struggle to fight it off in attempt to get better. This tends to exhaust a person's energy reserves and causes them to lose heart more easily, than if they simply settle into it and allow treatments being taken, to do their job. I thought this was excellent advice and especially with the fact that this same Doctor had experienced that very same form of cancer he was advising the patient in regard to and he experienced full remission and is still living well, many years later.

My own Hashimoto's Thyroiditis disease hit me especially hard because of the timing of the onset being at an extremely stressful and busy period of my life. It affected me greatly both physically and emotionally and I found it very hard to even accept that I had this disease.

I found after diagnosis years ago, that it would also require treatment, taking replacement hormone pills, likely for the rest of my life and this too was very hard for me to accept.

Like anyone else, I instead wanted a quick-fix for the problem, some way to overcome it and get rid of the disease – to eradicate it from my body. I found it very difficult to even reserve myself to taking the permanent, daily medication and in the back of my mind; I wanted to believe the Doctors were all wrong and that it was an incorrect diagnosis. I went on like this for the first several months and just as the Osteopath Doctor described, it caused a lot of frustration to build in me and I found myself getting exhausted from all of the worry and stress I was allowing myself to experience.

At one point, it occurred to me that it was possible that if I learned all I could about this disease, I might find all possible avenues for helping to cope with it and possibly even overcome it in my life. This was for me, part of embracing the disease because my wanting to learn all I could about it was part of the aspect of acceptance that needed to take place.

The internet is an incredible resource of information for any subject and is true of medical information as well, when obtained through reputable sources. No one should ever be discouraged from educating their selves about a disease they have but should of course study only that information that is reliable, such as that found on the more mainstream sources. You should study medical information on your disease, carefully and slowly and compare the information together with many reliable resources, so that correct information you find, is strongly confirmed. Your doctor should be willing to go over any information with you and answer questions as well.

I also realized at one point that I could learn from other patients who had my same disease and so I began to read on thyroid disease and hypothyroidism forums and message boards. This was another step in my embracing the disease rather than experiencing the negative effects of attempting to constantly struggle against it. After reading on many of these forums, I eventually registered as a member on some of them and began to correspond with other patients.

This came as a great comfort to me because patients many times feel very alone and isolated when they experience the onset of a disease and by finding others who have the same disease, whom they can correspond with, they no longer feel as alone with it.

For many of us, the steps toward accepting and embracing our disease, has helped us to become "thyroid patient advocates" for others suffering the same diseases. This acceptance and embracing only means we are doing so for the time-being, all the while our hopes being that better and more effective treatments are being developed and that medical science finds ways to conquer more and more of these chronic diseases. Many of us are also willing and open to divine intervention, if we believe in a higher power that can perform supernatural healing and I certainly do. We only accept the disease, so that we can learn about it for the time-being and this also helps take much of the fear out of it for us as well.

You do not fight and struggle against something you accept and embrace. Continual struggle against something you do not have complete control over by your natural, human powers, will cause frustration, fear and exhaustion.

Improving Life for Thyroid Patients

In reality, our only option until remission, cure or supernatural healing takes place, is to accept and embrace our disease and in the mean time, allow our treatments work their intended purposes.

Thyroid diseases can cause an array of diverse and life-changing symptoms. One aspect of coping for patients is learning to find acceptance for their disease as previously mentioned.

Some people who experience the onset of hypothyroid or hyperthyroid disorders find difficulty coping with a health disorder that in most cases requires lifelong treatment. A degree of change in one's ability to carry on with the same level of activities can diminish, causing a thyroid patient to feel disabled to some degree. These type changes can affect a patient emotionally, possibly requiring therapy to help them cope.

Administered Therapies and Self-Therapy

One aspect of emotional therapy that can help patients cope with thyroid disease is one in the "Cognitive Behavioral Therapy" category in which patients learn to react differently to changes thyroid symptoms may cause them.

This would be the goal rather than reacting negatively so that a patient can learn instead, to react with acceptance for something they have no power to change.

Thyroid disease treatments can help tremendously with relief of hormone-imbalance related symptoms but in most cases do not take away certain disease aspects and for some patients a need for coping therapies may arise. Therapy can be administered by mental health professionals in serious cases of emotional coping needs or as self-therapy in patients who have mild to moderate coping needs.

Changes That May Require Emotional Coping

While the general symptoms of thyroid disorders are not always significantly life-changing, others are more severe and can have an emotional impact on patients in a number of ways as previously mentioned. Women for example who develop thyroid autoimmunity, are sometimes required to delay pregnancies if they have highly elevated auto-antibody levels and some experience miscarriages due to this problem with autoimmunity.

Other thyroid patients develop Thyroid Eye Disease, in which their eyes bulge and protrude and they can remain in this condition for several years. Others experience significant hair loss or emotional symptoms that can be difficult to resolve and all of these scenarios can be difficult for affected patients to cope with in some cases.

Struggle Increases Stress

The "acceptance" aspect of learning to cope with thyroid disease is similar in-principle to CBT anxiety disorder therapies that teach anxiety sufferers not to struggle with anxiety but to simply learn to flow with it and allow it to take place. In the case of anxiety, continually struggling against symptoms simply fuels them because the "fight or flight" anxiety mechanism thrives on struggle, which serves to repeatedly reactivate them.

The same can be said of patients who struggle against a disease they have no control over, rather than learning to accept it as having become a part of their lives. This type acceptance in the case of a thyroid patient does not mean that he welcomes the disease or approves of it.

ans he accepts the fact that it has
ife and will remain there unless cured
or healed by divine intervention. By strongly
resisting a disease with ongoing mental and
physical struggle, a patient can actually increase
symptoms of stress, anxiety and fatigue.

Giving One's Self Permission to Feel Unwell

A thyroid patient must give himself permission to
feel sick if symptoms flare and permission to take
extra time to rest and relax. This might also
require upfront honesty with friends and relatives
who ask for his attendance at events he may not
feel able to attend. Simply being honest and
saying that the timing is not good for him can
help relieve the stress of expectations.

In most cases people understand when you
explain your reasons to them while others may
not be. Regardless, health and well being must
always come before pleasing others and a thyroid
patient cannot afford to add unnecessary stressors
to his life. This same advice can be applied to
patients suffering illnesses such as Chronic
Fatigue Syndrome and Fibromyalgia.

Medical studies have shown that chronic stress can directly affect thyroid disease severity. In addition to the described CBT coping methods, there are other psychiatric therapies that can help emotionally struggling thyroid patients, as well as medications that can be prescribed by their doctors.

It is my hope that the preceding chapters have provided inspiration to those who read them and helpful suggestions for improving the lives of thyroid disease patients.

(END)

www.ingramcontent.com/pod-product-compliance
Lightning Source LLC
Chambersburg PA
CBHW020348290526
45785CB00005B/2185